DEMYSTIFYING THE PIP PROCESS:

A Simplified Guide to Understanding and Applying for Beginners

MJ Blake

MJ BLAKE

TABLE OF CONTENTS

<u>DISCLAIMER</u>

The information provided in this book, "Demystifying the PIP Process: A Simplified Guide to Understanding and Applying for Beginners," is intended for general guidance purposes only. While every effort has been made to ensure the accuracy and completeness of the information, it is subject to change and may not cover all possible scenarios or individual circumstances.

This book is not a substitute for professional advice, and the author and publisher cannot be held responsible for any errors, omissions, or actions taken based on the information provided. Readers are encouraged to consult with qualified professionals, such as welfare rights advisors or legal experts, for personalized guidance and assistance related to their specific situations.

The Personal Independence Payment (PIP) process is subject to government regulations and policies, which may evolve over time. It is advisable to refer to the latest official sources, such as government websites or official publications, for the most up-to-date information.

The experiences and examples provided in this book are for illustrative purposes only and should not be taken as guaranteed outcomes or indicative of all PIP assessments or decisions. Each application is evaluated on an individual basis, and outcomes may vary depending on various factors.

Furthermore, the author and publisher disclaim any liability for any loss or damage, directly or indirectly, resulting from the use of this book or the application of the information provided herein. Readers are responsible for their own decisions and actions, and they should exercise caution and discretion when interpreting and applying the information in this book.

By reading this book, readers acknowledge that they understand and accept the limitations and disclaimers stated above.

MJ BLAKE

<u>ACKNOWLEDGMENT</u>

I would like to express my heartfelt gratitude to everyone who contributed to the creation of this book, "Demystifying the PIP Process: A Simplified Guide to Understanding and Applying for Beginners."

First and foremost, I extend my deepest appreciation to the individuals who shared their personal experiences and insights, allowing me to gain a deeper understanding of the challenges and intricacies of the PIP process. Your stories have been invaluable in shaping the content of this book and making it relatable to readers.

I would like to thank the welfare rights advisors, legal experts, and professionals who provided their expertise and guidance throughout the development of this book. Your knowledge and insights have helped ensure the accuracy and reliability of the information presented. Your dedication to supporting individuals navigating the PIP process is truly commendable.

A special thanks goes to the team at the publishing house for their assistance and support in bringing this book to life. Your professionalism, expertise, and commitment to delivering a high-quality publication have been instrumental in making this project a reality.

I am grateful to my friends and family for their unwavering encouragement, understanding, and belief in me throughout this writing journey. Your support has been a constant source of motivation, and I am truly grateful for your presence in my life.

Lastly, I would like to express my appreciation to the readers of this book. Your interest and willingness to explore the PIP process with an open mind inspire me. I hope that this guide serves as a valuable resource and empowers you to navigate the PIP application process with confidence and clarity.

While every effort has been made to provide accurate and helpful information, I welcome any feedback or suggestions for improvement. Together, we can continue to enhance the understanding and accessibility of the PIP process for individuals who need it the most.

Thank you all for being a part of this journey.

Sincerely, MJ Blake

MJ BLAKE

<u>DEDICATION</u>

This book is dedicated to all the individuals who have faced the challenges of the Personal Independence Payment (PIP) process.

To those who have struggled to understand the complexities and intricacies of the application, assessment, and decision-making processes, this book is for you. May it provide you with clarity, guidance, and the confidence to navigate the PIP journey.

To the resilient individuals who have courageously shared their stories, experiences, and insights, your contributions have made this book possible. Your voices have given life to the pages within, and your determination has inspired the creation of a resource that aims to support and empower others.

To the tireless advocates, welfare rights advisors, and professionals who work tirelessly to support individuals in their pursuit of PIP, thank you for your dedication and commitment. Your expertise, guidance, and unwavering support are invaluable in helping individuals access the support they deserve.

To the friends and family members who have provided unwavering love, understanding, and encouragement throughout the writing process, your support has been the foundation upon which this book stands. Your belief in the importance of helping others has fueled my determination to create a resource that simplifies and demystifies the PIP process.

Finally, to the readers of this book, may it serve as a beacon of hope and a source of knowledge. May it empower you to navigate the PIP process with confidence, ensuring that your needs are recognized and supported. Your journey is important, and I am honored to be a part of it.

With heartfelt gratitude and dedication,

MJ Blake

15

<u>PREFACE</u>

Welcome to "Demystifying the PIP Process: A Simplified Guide to Understanding and Applying for Beginners." This book aims to provide clear and accessible information about the Personal Independence Payment (PIP) process, designed specifically for individuals who are new to this complex system.

Navigating the PIP process can be overwhelming, with its forms, assessments, and eligibility criteria. The purpose of this guide is to demystify PIP and empower you with the knowledge and understanding you need to confidently engage with the application process.

Throughout the pages of this book, we will delve into the various aspects of PIP, breaking down the process into manageable steps and explaining key concepts in simplistic terms. Whether you are applying for PIP for the first time or seeking to understand the intricacies of the process, this guide is designed to be your companion, providing you with a roadmap to successfully navigate the PIP journey.

Drawing on research, expert insights, and real-life experiences, we have endeavored to create a comprehensive resource that covers the essential information you need to know. From understanding the purpose of PIP and its eligibility criteria to providing guidance on completing the application form, gathering supporting evidence, and preparing for the assessment, each chapter is crafted to address your concerns and questions.

It is important to note that the information contained in this guide is based on the knowledge available at the time of writing. The PIP process may undergo changes and updates over time, and it is advisable to refer to official sources for the most up-to-date information. However, the core principles and concepts discussed in this book will provide you with a solid foundation to approach the PIP process confidently and make informed decisions.

It is our sincere hope that this guide will empower you to understand the PIP process and navigate it successfully. We believe that everyone should have access to the support they need to live a fulfilling and independent life, and it is our mission to contribute to that goal by providing you with the knowledge and tools to engage effectively with the PIP system.

We encourage you to read this guide with an open mind, ask questions, and seek further support if needed. Remember, you are not alone in this journey. Many individuals have traveled the path before you, and many organizations and professionals are dedicated to supporting you throughout the process.

Thank you for choosing "Demystifying the PIP Process: A Simplified Guide to Understanding and Applying for Beginners." We are honored to be a part of your journey toward a better understanding of the PIP process, and we wish you success in your pursuit of the support you deserve.

19

<u>INTRODUCTION</u>

The title of this book is "Demystifying the PIP Process: A Simplified Guide to Understanding and Applying for Beginners." This manual will help you understand and apply for PIP. This book is a thorough resource that has been carefully designed to give readers who are unfamiliar with the Personal Independence Payment (PIP) application procedure a straightforward and approachable route to comprehending the application and successfully navigating it.

Applying for PIP can be challenging, especially if the applicant is not familiar with the nuances of the application process. By giving you the theoretical foundation and practical instructions required to successfully complete the Personal Injury Protection (PIP) application process, this guide aims to fill that knowledge gap.

Whether you are making an application on your own behalf or on behalf of a loved one, you can rely on this book to be a reliable reference. By breaking the PIP method down into more manageable parts and employing less technical terminology, we have made a concentrated attempt to explain the more complicated components in a way that is understandable. Our objective is to demystify PIP so that beginners can use it more easily.

The essentials of PIP, including its goal, prerequisites for eligibility, and the extensive application process's various elements, will be covered in the pages that follow. You will learn about the evaluation procedure, the significance of supporting documentation, and quick application form completion advice. We strive to give you the assurance and knowledge required to effectively navigate the PIP journey by answering some of the most frequently asked questions and concerns.

We make an effort to offer advice that may be used in a wide range of scenarios since we understand that each person's experiences are unique. By offering practical hints, examples from the real world, and guidance from experts in the field, we will give you a thorough knowledge of the procedures in this book.

Although this book offers helpful insights and practical solutions, it is not meant to replace professional guidance. To get customized support catered to your unique needs and circumstances, we strongly suggest you speak with welfare rights counsellors or attorneys. To stay up to date on the most recent developments, it is vital to consult official sources because government legislation and policies that apply to the PIP procedure are susceptible to change over time.

At the time of publication, we want to make sure that all the material in this book is correct and up to date. Despite this, we are aware that changes could be made to the PIP procedure and that new information might become available. Keep a proactive attitude, seek out new information as needed, and modify your plan as appropriate.

Regardless of where you are in the PIP application process or if you want to have a better grasp of the process, "Demystifying the PIP Process: A Simplified Guide to Understanding and Applying for Beginners" is here to help. We have great hopes that this manual will give you the knowledge and abilities required to successfully navigate the

PIP procedure and secure the support you require.

I'm glad you decided to make this book your main source of information. We are honored to help you understand and effectively complete the PIP procedure, and we salute your dedication to doing so.

MJ BLAKE

<u>1: THE PIP PROCESS</u>

In this chapter, we will provide an overview of the PIP process and its significance in supporting individuals with disabilities or long-term health conditions. We will delve into the key concepts, eligibility criteria, and the impact of PIP on daily life. By the end of this chapter, you will have a clear understanding of why PIP exists and who it is intended to help.

PIP, introduced in 2013, is a non-means-tested benefit provided by the Department for Work and Pensions (DWP) in the United Kingdom. It is designed to assist individuals aged between 16 and State Pension age who face challenges in carrying out daily activities or have difficulty getting around due to a health condition or disability.

We will explore the key components of PIP, namely the daily living and mobility components, and explain how they contribute to determining the level of support an individual may receive. By familiarizing yourself with these components, you will be better prepared to comprehend the assessment criteria and communicate your needs effectively during the application process.

Understanding the eligibility criteria is crucial, and we will discuss the specific requirements that applicants must meet to qualify for PIP. We will outline the general rules related to residence, age, and existing benefits, as well as delve into the specific descriptors that assessors use to determine the level of support an applicant may be eligible for.

Moreover, we will explore the potential impact of PIP on other benefits or services an individual may already receive. It is essential to understand how PIP interacts with other benefits to ensure that applicants can make informed decisions about their applications without risking any unintended consequences.

Throughout this chapter, we will strive to explain complex terms and concepts using simple language, ensuring that readers who are unfamiliar with the PIP process can grasp the information easily. By the end of this chapter, you will have a solid foundation in understanding the PIP process and be ready to delve deeper into the subsequent chapters that focus on the application process itself.

Remember, the aim of this book is to demystify the PIP process and empower you with the knowledge and confidence needed to apply for PIP. Let's embark on this journey together and unlock the doors to the support you or someone you know may be entitled to.

2: UNDERSTANDING THE APPLICATION REQUIREMENTS

In the following section, we will go deeper into the exact application requirements for the process of obtaining a Personal Independence Payment (PIP). It is critical that you have a solid understanding of these requirements so that you can increase the likelihood that your application will be accepted by providing information that is both true and pertinent. In this section, we will go over the application form in great detail, explaining and guiding you through each individual component as we go.

1. Personal Information: You will be asked for personal information in the first section of the PIP application form, including your full name, address, date of birth, and National Insurance number. Make sure the data you provide is accurate because any errors could potentially cause more delays or

problems during the evaluation process. Make sure you have their permission before applying on someone else's behalf and that the data you provide about them is accurate.

2. Contact Details: In this section, you will be asked to provide contact details, such as your phone number and email address. It's crucial to provide up-to-date contact information to ensure effective communication with the Department for Work and Pensions (DWP) throughout the application process. If your contact details change after submitting the application, inform the DWP as soon as possible.

3. Current Benefits and Employment Details: This section requires you to provide details about any existing benefits or employment. You will need to disclose information about the benefits you are currently receiving, such as Employment and Support Allowance (ESA) or Universal Credit. Additionally, if you are employed, you will be asked to provide information about your job, including the hours you

work and any adaptations or support you receive at work.

4. Healthcare Professionals Involved: Here, you will be asked to provide details of any healthcare professionals who have been involved in your care. This includes doctors, specialists, therapists, or any other professionals who have diagnosed or treated your condition. It's important to list all relevant healthcare professionals and provide their contact information, as the DWP may reach out to them for further information during the assessment process.

5. Medications and Treatments: This section requires you to provide information about any medications or treatments you are currently undergoing. Include the names of the medications, dosages, and the healthcare professional who prescribed them. If you have any medical equipment or aids that you use regularly, make sure to mention them as well. Providing accurate and detailed information about your treatments and medications will help

assessors understand the impact of your condition on your daily life.

6. Daily Living Activities: Understanding how your health impacts your capacity to carry out daily living activities is one of the PIP assessment's key components. You will be asked to answer questions in this section about a variety of activities, including meal preparation and cooking, medication management, dressing and undressing, washing and bathing, using the bathroom, and partaking in social events. Describe any difficulties or issues you encounter when carrying out these activities in detail, using concrete instances.

7. Mobility Activities: The mobility component of PIP focuses on your ability to get around. In this section, you will be asked about your mobility needs, including whether you require aids such as a wheelchair or mobility scooter. You will also need to provide information about any difficulties you face when navigating different environments, such as walking short or long distances, using

public transportation, or planning and following a journey.

8. Additional Information: In the final section of the application form, you will have the opportunity to provide any additional information or explanations that you believe are relevant to your application. This is your chance to expand on specific challenges, limitations, or circumstances that may not have been covered in the previous sections. Take advantage of this space to provide a comprehensive overview of your condition and its impact on your daily life.

Remember, when completing the PIP application form, it's crucial to be honest, thorough, and provide accurate information. Take your time to ensure that you understand each section and provide detailed responses. If you need assistance, consider reaching out to relevant support organizations or seeking guidance from a welfare rights advisor.

By understanding and meeting the application requirements, you lay a solid foundation for a successful PIP application. In the next chapter, we will explore the process of preparing for the PIP application, including gathering supporting documents and evidence to strengthen your case.

3: PREPARING FOR THE PIP APPLICATION

We will walk you through the process of getting ready for your Personal Independence Payment (PIP) application in this chapter. A thorough and accurate presentation of your disease and how it affects your daily life depends on your level of preparedness. You will be well-prepared to submit a powerful and well-supported application if you adhere to the procedures provided in this chapter.

1. Understand the PIP Criteria: Before you begin preparing your application, it's essential to have a clear understanding of the eligibility criteria and how PIP assessments are conducted. Familiarize yourself with the descriptors used by assessors to determine the level of support you may be entitled to. Review the PIP assessment criteria and make note of how your condition aligns with these criteria. This will help you gather the necessary evidence and provide relevant examples in your application.

2. Gather Supporting Documents: Collecting supporting documents is an important step in preparing for your PIP application. These documents serve as evidence to substantiate the information provided in your application. Examples of supporting documents include medical records, diagnosis reports, specialist letters, prescriptions, and any other relevant documents related to your condition. Contact your healthcare professionals and request copies of your medical records and any supporting documents they can provide. Ensure that these documents are up to date and accurately reflect your current situation.

3. Seek Supporting Statements: In addition to medical documents, obtaining supporting statements from professionals who are familiar with your condition can significantly strengthen your application. Consider reaching out to your healthcare providers, including doctors, specialists, therapists, or social workers, and request written statements that outline the impact of your condition on your daily life. These statements should highlight specific

examples and provide insights into the challenges you face. Ensure that the statements are signed and dated by the professionals, as this adds credibility to your application.

4. Document Your Daily Challenges: To present a comprehensive picture of how your condition affects your daily life, it's crucial to document the specific challenges you face. Keep a diary or journal where you can record the difficulties you encounter in performing daily living activities or getting around. Note down instances where you require assistance, experience pain or discomfort, or face limitations due to your condition. These detailed accounts will help you provide accurate and specific information in your application, reinforcing the impact of your condition on your day-to-day functioning.

5. Prepare Detailed Examples: When completing the application form, providing detailed examples that illustrate the challenges you face is vital. Think about specific instances where your

condition has hindered your ability to carry out activities. Describe the impact on your physical or mental well-being, any pain or discomfort experienced, and the assistance required. Use these examples to provide a clear and vivid picture of how your condition affects your ability to live independently and participate in society.

6. Organize Your Information: To streamline the application process, it's crucial to organize your information effectively. Create separate folders or sections for different types of documents, such as medical records, supporting statements, and any other relevant paperwork. Develop a system that allows you to easily access the information you need while completing the application form. Being organized not only saves time but also ensures that you don't overlook any critical documents or information during the application process.

7. Review and Double-Check: Before submitting your application, carefully review all the information you have

provided. Ensure that you have answered all the questions accurately and thoroughly. Double-check your supporting documents to confirm that they are up to date and include all relevant information. Review your examples and statements to ensure they accurately reflect your experiences and challenges. Taking the time to review and double-check your application will help minimize errors or omissions and increase your chances of a successful outcome.

By following these steps and adequately preparing for your PIP application, you will be well-prepared to present a compelling case that accurately reflects the impact of your condition on your daily life. In the next chapter, we will guide you through the process of navigating the PIP application form itself, providing tips and explanations for each section.

4: NAVIGATING THE PIP APPLICATION FORM

In this chapter, we will guide you through the process of completing the Personal Independence Payment (PIP) application form. The application form can seem daunting at first glance, but by breaking it down into sections and understanding the purpose of each section, you will be better equipped to navigate through it successfully.

- Section 1: Personal Details – The first section of the PIP application form requires you to provide your personal information, such as your name, address, date of birth, and National Insurance number. Ensure that you provide accurate information and double-check for any errors. If you are completing the form on behalf of someone else, provide their details accurately and include your own contact information for correspondence.

- Section 2: Contact Details – In this section, you will provide your contact details, including your phone number and email address. Make sure to provide up-to-date contact information as the Department for Work and Pensions (DWP) may need to communicate with you during the assessment process. If your contact details change after submitting the application, inform the DWP as soon as possible to avoid any communication issues.

- Section 3: Current Benefits and Employment Details – This section requires you to provide details about any existing benefits you receive, such as Employment and Support Allowance (ESA) or Universal Credit. If you are employed, you will also need to provide information about your job, including the hours you work and any adaptations or support you receive at work. Be thorough in providing accurate information about your current benefits and employment status.

- Section 4: Participating Healthcare Professionals – You will be required to provide details on the medical personnel who have assisted in your care in this section. Identify the doctors, specialists, therapists, and/or other health care providers who diagnosed or treated your problem, together with their names and contact information. By providing their information, you enable the DWP to contact you for more information or clarification if necessary throughout the assessment process.

- Section 5: Medications and Treatments – This section requires you to provide details about any medications or treatments you are currently undergoing. Include the names of the medications, dosages, and the healthcare professional who prescribed them. If you use medical equipment or aids, mention them as well. Providing accurate and comprehensive information about your medications and treatments helps assessors understand the impact of your condition on your daily life.

- Section 6: Activities of Daily Life – The PIP assessment's main focus area is on how your condition impacts your capacity to perform daily life activities. You will be asked to answer questions in this section about a variety of tasks, including food preparation and cooking, managing medications, dressing and undressing, washing and bathing, using the bathroom, and participating in social events. Take your time when answering and be sure to include specific examples and any challenges you encountered when carrying out these tasks.

- Section 7: Mobility Activities The mobility component of PIP assesses your ability to get around. In this section, you will be asked about your mobility needs, such as whether you require aids like a wheelchair or mobility scooter. You will also need to provide information about any difficulties you face when navigating different environments, such as walking short or long distances, using public transportation, or planning and following a journey. Be specific in describing the challenges you encounter and how they impact your mobility.

- Section 8: Additional Information – The final section of the application form provides an opportunity to include any additional information or explanations that you believe are relevant to your application. Use this section to expand on specific challenges, limitations, or circumstances that may not have been covered in the previous sections. Provide any other relevant details that support your case and give a comprehensive understanding of your condition and its impact on your daily life.

Throughout the form, it's crucial to be honest, provide accurate information, and use specific examples to illustrate the challenges you face. Take your time to read each question carefully and consider how it relates to your condition. Seek assistance from support organizations or welfare rights advisors if needed to ensure that you complete the form accurately and effectively.

Once you have completed the application form, review it thoroughly for any errors or omissions. Ensure that all sections are filled out accurately and that you have provided supporting documents where necessary. By carefully navigating the PIP application form, you will be one step closer to submitting a comprehensive and compelling application.

In the next chapter, we will discuss the importance of gathering supporting evidence and how to present it effectively to strengthen your PIP application.

5: SUPPORTING DOCUMENTS AND EVIDENCE

We will discuss the relevance of assembling supporting paperwork and proof for your Personal Independence Payment (PIP) application in this chapter. It's crucial to back up your assertions with solid, pertinent information that shows how your ailment affects your daily life. You may boost your PIP application by being aware of the kinds of supporting papers you can collect and how to present them well.

1. Medical Records and Diagnosis Reports: Your medical records are one of the most important pieces of proof. These papers give a full picture of your health state and its history. Get copies of your medical information from your doctors, specialists, and therapists by contacting them. Diagnose reports, treatment plans, notes on how the treatment is going, and any other important medical information should be in these records. Make sure your medical records are accurate and up to date with your present health.

2. Specialist Letters and Reports: If you have received treatment or consultations from specialists, such as consultants or therapists, consider requesting letters or reports from them. These documents provide expert opinions on your condition and can help demonstrate the severity and impact of your symptoms. Specialist letters should include information about your diagnosis, the nature of your condition, any limitations or challenges you face, and recommendations for support or treatment.

3. Supporting Statements from Healthcare Professionals: Obtaining supporting statements from healthcare professionals who are familiar with your condition can be highly beneficial. These statements should be written by professionals who have treated or assessed you, such as doctors, therapists, or social workers. The statements should highlight the specific impact of your condition on your daily life, providing detailed examples and insights into the challenges you face. Ensure that the statements are signed, dated, and include the professional's

contact information for verification if
needed.

4. Prescriptions and Medication Information:
Including information about your
prescribed medications and treatments
can provide further evidence of the
impact of your condition. Make a list of
the medications you take, including the
names, dosages, and frequencies. Include
any side effects or limitations caused by
the medications. Additionally, if you use
medical equipment or aids, such as
mobility aids or assistive devices, include
information about them as well.

5. Care Plans or Documents of Support: If
you get care or support services, like
home care or help from carers, including
relevant care plans or documents of
support can help your application. These
papers explain the specific help you need
and show how much help you need with
things you do every day. They can give
you a clear picture of the problems you're
facing and the help you need to stay
independent.

6. Letters from Employers or Educational Institutions: If you work or go to school, you might want to get letters from your workplace or school. These letters can talk about any changes that were made at your job or school to help you. They can also help you understand how your condition affects your ability to do jobs or fully participate in work or school.

7. Personal Statements and Diaries: In addition to official documents, personal statements and diaries can be powerful pieces of evidence. Write a personal statement where you describe your experiences, challenges, and limitations due to your condition. Use specific examples to illustrate the impact on your daily life. Keeping a diary or journal where you document your symptoms, difficulties, and the support you require can also be valuable evidence. Include dates, times, and details of each entry to provide a comprehensive account of your condition.

8. Relevant Photographs or Videos: In some cases, including photographs or videos

can visually demonstrate the challenges you face. For example, if you require aids or adaptations in your home or if you experience visible physical symptoms, capturing them through photographs or videos can be impactful evidence. Ensure that the visuals are clear and accurately represent your situation.

When submitting supporting documents and evidence, it's essential to organize them effectively. Label each document clearly and provide a summary or index to help assessors navigate through the information. Include a cover letter that outlines the supporting documents you have included and briefly explains their relevance to your application.

Remember to make copies of all the documents you submit and keep them for your records. This will help you reference the information if needed and ensure that you have a comprehensive record of your application.

In the next chapter, we will discuss how to present your information effectively on the PIP application form itself, including tips on structuring your answers and providing relevant examples.

6: TIPS FOR A SUCCESSFUL PIP APPLICATION

In this chapter, we will provide you with valuable tips and strategies to maximize your chances of a successful Personal Independence Payment (PIP) application. By following these guidelines and incorporating them into your application, you can enhance the clarity, accuracy, and persuasiveness of your submission.

- Understand the PIP Criteria: To ensure a successful application, it's crucial to have a clear understanding of the eligibility criteria and how the PIP assessment process works. Familiarize yourself with the descriptors used by assessors to determine the level of support you may be entitled to. This understanding will help you gather the necessary evidence and provide relevant examples that align with the criteria.

- Be Clear and Specific: When completing the application form, strive for clarity and specificity in your answers. Clearly explain how your condition affects your daily life and provide specific examples to illustrate the challenges you face. Avoid using vague or generalized statements. Instead, focus on providing detailed accounts of your limitations, difficulties, and the support you require. The more precise and detailed your responses, the better assessors can understand the impact of your condition.

- Link Your Condition to PIP Descriptors: Make explicit connections between your condition and the descriptors used in the PIP assessment. Consider how your symptoms align with each descriptor and provide relevant evidence to support your claims. Ensure that you address each relevant descriptor and provide examples that clearly demonstrate how your condition meets the criteria. This will strengthen your case and increase your chances of a successful outcome.

- Focus on Functionality and Daily Living Activities: The PIP assessment mainly looks at how your health affects your ability to do daily living activities and move around. When filling out the application form and giving proof, stress how your condition affects your ability to work and live on your own. Describe in detail the problems you have with things like taking care of yourself, making meals, taking care of your medications, moving around, and talking to people. Give detailed examples and talk about the help you need to do these things.

- Include Relevant Supporting Evidence: Gather and include all relevant supporting evidence with your application. This includes medical records, diagnosis reports, specialist letters, prescriptions, care plans, and any other documents that substantiate your claims. Ensure that the evidence is up to date and accurately reflects your current condition. Clearly label each document and provide a summary or index to help assessors navigate through the information effectively.

- Provide Comprehensive and Consistent Information: Ensure that the information you provide in your application form, supporting documents, and personal statements is consistent and comprehensive. Avoid contradictions or inconsistencies that may raise doubts about the accuracy of your claims. Review all the information before submitting your application to ensure that it presents a coherent and accurate representation of your condition and its impact.

- Use Clear and Easy-to-Understand Language: Use clear and easy-to-understand language when filling out the application form and giving answers. Don't use jargon or scientific terms that the reader may not know. Instead, use simple words to talk about your situation, its symptoms, and what you can't do. This will make it easier for assessors to get a clear picture of your position.

- Seek Support and Guidance: If you feel overwhelmed or unsure about completing the PIP application, seek support and guidance from relevant organizations or welfare rights advisors. They can provide assistance in understanding the process, reviewing your application, and offering valuable insights. These professionals are experienced in PIP applications and can help ensure that your application is comprehensive and well-prepared.

- Keep a Copy of Your Application: Make a copy of your completed application form and all supporting documents for your records. This will serve as a reference point in case any issues arise during the assessment process or if you need to provide additional information later. Having a copy of your application ensures that you have a comprehensive record of the information you submitted.

- Be Honest and Accurate: Above all, be honest and accurate in your application. Provide a true and transparent account of your condition and its impact on your daily life. Exaggerating or downplaying your symptoms may compromise the credibility of your application. Assessors are trained to identify inconsistencies, so it's crucial to provide an accurate representation of your circumstances.

By following these tips, you can enhance the quality and effectiveness of your PIP application. In the next chapter, we will discuss what to expect after submitting your application, including the assessment process, potential outcomes, and steps to take if you disagree with the decision.

7: THE ASSESSMENT PROCESS EXPLAINED

In this chapter, we will guide you through the assessment process for Personal Independence Payment (PIP). Once you have submitted your application, it will undergo a thorough assessment to determine your eligibility for PIP and the level of support you may be entitled to. Understanding the assessment process will help you navigate through it confidently and provide any necessary additional information or clarification.

1. Application Review: After submitting your PIP application, it will be reviewed by the Department for Work and Pensions (DWP). During this initial stage, they will check if all the required information and supporting documents have been provided. If any essential information is missing, the DWP may contact you to request additional details or documentation. It's important to respond promptly and provide the requested

information to avoid delays in the assessment process.

2. Consultation with Healthcare Professional: In most cases, the next step in the assessment process involves a consultation with a healthcare professional. The purpose of this consultation is to gather further information about your condition and how it affects your daily life. The healthcare professional may be a doctor, nurse, or occupational therapist trained in conducting PIP assessments. They will assess your functional abilities based on the PIP criteria and ask you questions about your condition and the impact it has on various aspects of your life.

3. Functionality and Capability Assessment: During the assessment, the medical professional will look at how well you can do daily living chores and move around. They will look at the information you gave them in your application and during the meeting to figure out how your condition affects your ability to do certain things. The healthcare worker will look at the PIP

descriptors and give you points based on how much help you may be able to get.

4. Supporting Evidence Consideration: The healthcare professional will also review the supporting evidence you submitted with your application. This includes medical records, specialist letters, and any other relevant documents. The evidence will be taken into account during the assessment to support the conclusions drawn by the healthcare professional. It is crucial to ensure that the supporting evidence accurately reflects your condition and its impact on your daily life.

5. Assessment Report and Decision: Based on the information gathered during the consultation and the review of supporting evidence, the healthcare professional will compile an assessment report. This report will include details of the assessment findings, the functional abilities observed, and the level of support recommended based on the PIP descriptors. The report will then be sent to the DWP for a final decision on your PIP claim.

6. Letter of Decision: Once the DWP has reviewed the assessment report, they will send you a letter informing you of their decision regarding your PIP claim. This letter will be sent to you once they have made their decision. In the letter of decision, the amount of any payout, if any, as well as the reasoning behind the decision, will be detailed. In the event that you qualify for PIP, the letter will also inform you of when it will begin and how long it will continue for. In the event that your claim is rejected, you will receive a letter that details the reasoning behind the decision as well as instructions on how to appeal the decision.

7. Award Review: It's important to note that PIP awards are not indefinite. The DWP periodically reviews PIP awards to ensure that they remain accurate and reflective of the claimant's circumstances. The review process may involve requesting updated information, conducting another assessment, or reassessing the claim based on existing evidence. It's essential to respond to any review requests promptly and provide accurate and up-

to-date information to avoid any disruption to your PIP award.

8. Challenging the Decision: If you disagree with the decision made regarding your PIP claim, you have the right to challenge it. The decision letter will provide information on how to request a mandatory reconsideration, which involves asking the DWP to review their decision. If the mandatory reconsideration does not change the decision, you can further appeal to an independent tribunal. Seek advice from support organizations or welfare rights advisors to understand the process and receive guidance on challenging the decision effectively.

By understanding the assessment process, you can better prepare for each stage and provide any necessary information or clarification. In the final chapter, we will conclude our guide with important tips for managing your PIP award, including reporting changes in circumstances and seeking support when needed.

8: <u>NEXT STEPS AFTER THE PIP DECISION</u>

In this final chapter, we will discuss the important steps to take after receiving a decision on your Personal Independence Payment (PIP) claim. Whether you have been awarded PIP or your claim has been unsuccessful, it's crucial to understand your rights and responsibilities, as well as the available support and resources.

1. Award Confirmation If your Personal Independence Payment (PIP) claim is approved, the Department of Work and Pensions (DWP) will send you a formal letter confirming that you have been approved for the payment. This letter will clarify the specifics of your PIP award, including the amount of support you will receive, when the award will begin, and how long it will last. Be sure to hide this letter somewhere secure and make duplicates of it for your files.

2. Understanding Your Award: Take the time to fully understand the terms and conditions of your PIP award. Familiarize yourself with the specific activities and descriptors for which you have been awarded points. This will help you recognize the areas where you are entitled to support and ensure that you receive the correct level of assistance.

3. Reporting Changes in Circumstances: It is essential to inform the DWP promptly if there are any changes in your circumstances that may affect your PIP award. This includes changes in your health condition, functional abilities, living arrangements, or financial situation. Failing to report changes may result in an overpayment or underpayment of your PIP. Contact the PIP helpline or submit a change of circumstances form to provide updated information.

4. Award Reviews: The DWP periodically reviews PIP awards to ensure that they remain accurate and reflect your current circumstances. If your award is subject to review, you will receive a letter requesting

updated information or inviting you to attend another assessment. Respond to these requests promptly and provide accurate and up-to-date information to ensure that your award remains appropriate.

5. Appealing an Unsuccessful Claim: If your PIP claim is unsuccessful or you disagree with the decision made, you have the right to appeal. The decision letter you receive will explain the process for requesting a mandatory reconsideration, which involves asking the DWP to review their decision. Provide additional evidence or clarification to support your case during the mandatory reconsideration stage. If the decision remains unchanged, you can further appeal to an independent tribunal. Seek advice and support from organizations specializing in welfare rights to navigate the appeals process effectively.

6. Seeking Additional Support: Managing your PIP award can sometimes be challenging, especially if your needs change or you require further support.

There are various resources and organizations available to provide assistance. Contact local support organizations, welfare rights advisors, or disability advocacy services for guidance and advice. They can help you access additional support, understand your rights, and provide assistance in dealing with any issues that may arise.

7. Maximizing your Entitlements: In addition to PIP, you may be eligible for other benefits or entitlements. Research and explore other financial support options, such as Universal Credit, Employment and Support Allowance (ESA), or Disability Living Allowance (DLA). Each benefit has its own eligibility criteria and application process, so ensure you understand the requirements and consider seeking advice from experts to determine which benefits you may be entitled to.

8. Self-Care and Well-being: Coping with a health condition or disability can be physically and emotionally challenging. It's essential to prioritize self-care and well-being. Seek support from healthcare

professionals, therapists, or support groups to manage your condition effectively. Take advantage of community services, respite care, or counseling services if needed. Remember that your well-being is paramount, and accessing the necessary support can significantly improve your quality of life.

By taking these next steps after the PIP decision, you can effectively manage your award, stay informed of your rights and responsibilities, and seek additional support when necessary. Remember that your circumstances may change, and it's important to stay proactive in maintaining accurate and up-to-date information.

9: PERSONAL STORIES OF THE PIP PROCESS FROM REAL PEOPLE

In this chapter, we will delve into the personal stories of individuals who have gone through the Personal Independence Payment (PIP) process. These stories aim to provide insight, empathy, and a deeper understanding of the challenges, triumphs, and lessons learned from real-life experiences. By sharing these narratives, we hope to shed light on the diverse journeys individuals have taken and offer encouragement to those currently navigating the PIP process.

Sarah's Journey: Overcoming Barriers and Advocating for Rights

Sarah's story begins with her initial confusion and anxiety when faced with the PIP application. She candidly shares her struggles in understanding the complex eligibility criteria and how she overcame barriers through extensive research, seeking advice from welfare rights advisors, and connecting with support networks. Sarah's story highlights the importance of self-advocacy and persistence in navigating the PIP process.

David's Experience: Challenging Stereotypes and Obtaining a Fair Assessment

David, a young man with an invisible disability, recounts his journey of proving the impact of his condition on his daily life during the assessment stage. He shares the challenges he faced due to the lack of awareness and understanding of his condition, and the steps he took to educate and empower himself throughout the process. David's story emphasizes the need for increased awareness and understanding of invisible disabilities within the PIP system.

Emma's Battle: From Initial Rejection to Successful Appeal

Emma's story reflects her initial disappointment and frustration when her PIP application was rejected. She takes us through her journey of gathering additional evidence, seeking legal support, and navigating the appeals process. Emma's perseverance, coupled with the support of her legal representative, led to a successful appeal and a favorable outcome. Her story serves as a testament to the importance of persistence and seeking professional assistance when facing a setback.

Mark's Story: PIP Renewal and the Importance of Continual Documentation

Mark shares his experience of going through the PIP renewal process. He highlights the significance of maintaining ongoing documentation, gathering supporting evidence, and keeping track of changes in his condition and daily living needs. Mark's story emphasizes the importance of being proactive and prepared when it comes to PIP renewals, ensuring that the assessment accurately reflects the individual's current circumstances.

Laura's Journey: Navigating the PIP Process as a Carer

Laura's story offers a unique perspective as she recounts her experience as a carer supporting her father throughout the PIP application process. She shares the challenges faced, such as gathering evidence on behalf of her father and ensuring his needs were accurately represented. Laura's story highlights the vital role of carers in the PIP process and the need for adequate support and recognition of their contributions.

Conclusion

The personal stories shared in this chapter illuminate the human side of the PIP process. They reveal the triumphs, struggles, and resilience of individuals navigating the system.

Each story showcases the importance of perseverance, self-advocacy, seeking support, and staying informed throughout the journey. By listening to these real-life experiences, we gain valuable insights into the diverse challenges faced by individuals applying for PIP. Their stories inspire us to keep pushing for a more inclusive and understanding PIP system.

It is our hope that these personal narratives will provide comfort, guidance, and motivation to those currently going through the PIP process. May they remind you that you are not alone, and that there is strength in sharing experiences and learning from one another.

CONCLUSION

Congratulations on completing "Demystifying the PIP Process: A Simplified Guide to Understanding and Applying for Beginners."

You have reached the end of this comprehensive resource, and we hope that it has equipped you with the knowledge, confidence, and practical insights to navigate the Personal Independence Payment (PIP) process successfully.

Throughout this book, we have strived to simplify the complexities of the PIP process, providing you with a clear understanding of its purpose, eligibility criteria, application requirements, and assessment procedure.

We have delved into the importance of gathering supporting evidence, completing the application form accurately, and preparing for the assessment. By addressing common questions and concerns, we aimed to empower you to approach the PIP journey with greater clarity and readiness.

Remember, the information presented in this guide is accurate and up to date at the time of publication. However, the PIP process may evolve, and new developments may arise. We encourage you to stay informed about the latest updates through official sources and seek professional guidance when needed. The journey towards accessing the support you deserve may require ongoing learning and adaptation.

We want to emphasize the importance of advocating for yourself and seeking the support you need. The PIP process can be challenging, but with persistence, knowledge, and a proactive approach, you can navigate it successfully. You have the right to be heard, understood, and supported throughout this process.

We would like to express our sincere appreciation to you for choosing this book as your guide. Your commitment to understanding and navigating the PIP process demonstrates your determination to access the support that can make a positive difference in your life. We hope that this guide has provided you with the clarity and confidence to move forward.

Remember, you are not alone. There are professionals, organizations, and support networks available to assist you on your PIP journey. Reach out to welfare rights advisors, legal experts, or disability advocacy groups for additional guidance tailored to your unique circumstances.

As you continue your journey, we encourage you to remain resilient and persistent. Your voice matters, and you have the right to access the support you need to live a fulfilling and independent life. The road may have its challenges, but with the knowledge and insights gained from this guide, you are better equipped to face them.

Once again, we congratulate you on completing "Demystifying the PIP Process: A Simplified Guide to Understanding and Applying for Beginners." We hope that this book has provided you with valuable information, guidance, and encouragement. May it serve as a trusted resource as you navigate the PIP process and take steps towards securing the support you deserve.

Best wishes for a successful PIP journey and a brighter future ahead.

Sincerely, MJ Blake

ABOUT THE AUTHOR

MJ Blake is an advocate, author, and devoted mother who has been on a journey of growth and empowerment since her two children were diagnosed with ADHD and autism. Through her personal struggles, she has recognized the significance of advocating for her children, promoting awareness, and educating others.

Through her candid and empathetic voice, she motivates other families to persevere and continue advocating for their children.

Outside of writing, MJ relishes spending time with her loved ones and volunteering with organizations that support children with special needs. She is devoted to spreading awareness and encouraging families in similar circumstances to find hope and encouragement.

MJ BLAKE